Terry Bolin is a prom[...]
Associate Professor [...]
Wales and visiting physician at the Prince of Wales Hospital.

As President of The Gut Foundation, he has taken a leading role in educating the medical profession and the general public about a wide range of common gastrointestinal problems.

Terry is the author of over 50 scientific publications as well as two textbooks of medicine covering analysis of symptoms and diagnosis. His research publications include milk intolerance, peptic ulcer disease, interactions between infection and nutrition, persistent diarrhoea, constipation, liver disease and bowel cancer. This book reflects a long-standing interest in intestinal gas.

Rosemary Stanton is Australia's best-known nutritionist. This is her 15th book, including two nutrition textbooks, and she has published several thousand articles on nutrition in newspapers and magazines as well as writing many papers for scientific journals. She appears frequently on television and radio and specialises in translating complex nutrition information into an easily-digestible form. Rosemary is also a council member of The Gut Foundation.

In her consulting business, clients include State and Commonwealth government departments, sports associations and teams, selected sections of the food industry, advertising and public relations companies. She also lectures to medical students, doctors, nurses, teachers, executives, sporting groups and the general public.

Rosemary's major aim is to change Australia's poor eating habits so that we have healthier diets, and eat more enjoyable foods. She believes understanding the normal actions of the human intestine will help people feel more comfortable about eating the wonderful range of high fibre foods available.

WIND BREAKS

Coming to Terms with Wind

Terry Bolin
and
Rosemary Stanton

MARGARET
Gee

Published by
Margaret Gee Publishing
an imprint of
Margaret Gee Holdings
P.O. Box 221, Double Bay NSW 2028
A.C.N. 005 604 464

First published in 1993
Reprinted 1993, 1994

Distributed by Gary Allen Pty Ltd
9 Cooper Street, Smithfield NSW 2164

Copyright © Terry Bolin & Rosemary Stanton 1993
Cartoons copyright © Ron Tandberg 1993

All rights reserved. No part of this publication may be reproduced, stored in a retrieval system, or transmitted in any form or by any means electronic, mechanical, photocopying, recording or otherwise without the prior permission of the Publisher.

National Library of Australia
Cataloguing-in-Publication entry

Bolin, T.D. (Terry Dorcen).
  Wind breaks.

  Includes index.
  ISBN 1 875574 18 2.

  1. Gastrointestinal gas—Popular works. I. Stanton, Rosemary. II. Title.

612.3

Typeset in 10/14pt Caxton by Midland Typesetters, Victoria
Printed by McPherson's Printing Group, Victoria
Production by Vantage Graphics, Sydney

Foreword

When we mentioned to friends, colleagues and relatives that we were writing a book on intestinal gases, they looked at us with disbelief and amusement. A few were shocked. In a so-called enlightened society, we wonder why so many people find a completely normal bodily function so embarrassing. Most people are so shy about the subject that they won't even ask their doctor about it. Many will not follow a healthy diet because they find it produces more gas. Sellers of beans know their sales would soar if someone could find a way to deflate the anti-social reputation of these nutritious little packages.

Most people know little about the gas which they discharge many times a day. Some consider it abnormal to produce any gas at all! A few claim they never fart—a point almost always disputed by those who live with them!

From the medical point of view, most doctors know much less about human gaseous emissions than veterinarians know about the flatology of animals. Bovine bloat is well-researched and ruminants' methane production and its greenhouse effects attract worldwide attention. Sadly, most medical researchers do not find human gas an attractive or profitable area for research so few spend much time contemplating human flatal fate. More information on the subject, however, is slowly emerging.

In this book, we have tackled the subject of gas seriously, aiming to give answers to the questions our patients have asked us over the years. Where we do not have answers, we have said so. Because of our society's taboo on the whole area of flatus we have also included a few humorous quotes and cartoons to lighten the subject.

We hope you enjoy reading this book, and that it will help you understand more about your body's inner workings so you have fewer fears about matters gaseous. Like Hippocrates, we believe that 'passing gas is necessary to well-being'.

We are especially indebted to those same friends, colleagues and relatives who found it impossible to resist the invitation to participate in our study of normal flatus patterns.

Terry Bolin
Rosemary Stanton

The Digestive System

In the mouth

Digestion begins in the mouth as foods are chewed and mixed with saliva. Enzymes in saliva begin to break down some of the complex carbohydrates (also called 'starches'). Chewing food thoroughly is essential for good digestion. As you swallow food, you can also swallow air. If you eat quickly or when you are tense, you will swallow more air. Swallowing also starts muscular contractions moving food down the oesophagus to the stomach.

Passage down the oesophagus

At the lower end of the oesophagus there is a valve that controls movement of food into the stomach and prevents acid and the stomach contents from refluxing (coming back into the oesophagus). As we swallow, the valve relaxes so that food moves down into the stomach.

In the stomach

The cells lining the stomach produce acidic gastric juices which contain some enzymes to begin breaking down protein into smaller pieces. The mass of food in the stomach is churned by the stomach acid to a soupy consistency, ready to pass to the small intestine.

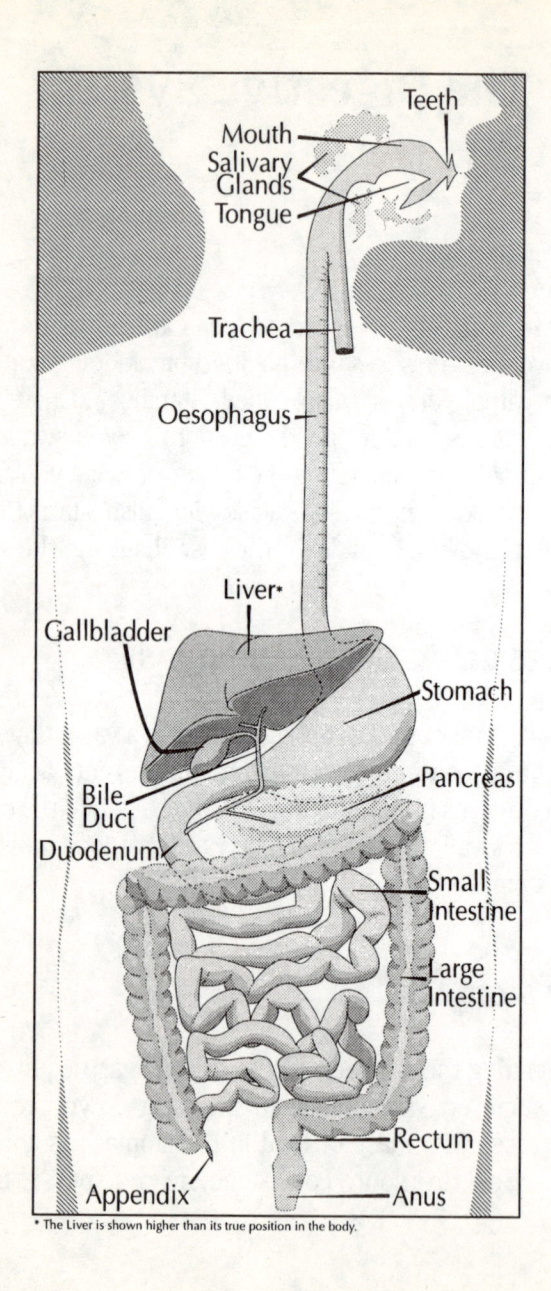

* The Liver is shown higher than its true position in the body.

Alcohol and some drugs can be absorbed directly from the stomach but most of the mass of food passes through to the small intestine. Carbohydrates eaten on their own tend to leave the stomach quickly. Proteins and fats delay the emptying of the stomach and so make you feel more satisfied after eating. If you consume large quantities of fat, the mass of food will take many hours to leave the stomach and may produce unpleasant feelings of 'fullness'.

It usually takes about four hours for the stomach to empty completely. Soon after the stomach is empty, you begin to feel hungry. The time taken for the stomach to empty corresponds to the usual human habit of eating three meals a day. Those who eat small meals will feel hungry more often.

In the small intestine

Most of the digestion of foods and the absorption of nutrients occurs in the small intestine. Here, juices from the pancreas neutralise the acid from the stomach. Enzymes from pancreatic juice and intestinal secretions break down carbohydrates, proteins and fats. The liver also produces bile which is stored in the gall bladder until it is needed in the small intestine to help digest fats.

Once the various food components have been digested in the small intestine, they are absorbed into the bloodstream and go to the liver. From the liver, the nutrients are distributed to the body and provide kilojoules of energy to all body cells. Dietary fibre, some sugars and some of the complex carbohydrates are not digested in the small intestine and pass to the large intestine.

It takes from 15 minutes to two hours for the first part of a meal to pass through the stomach and small intestine to reach the colon. The entire meal will take much longer. If, for some medical reason, transit through the stomach and small intestine is too rapid, less starch will be digested in the small intestine and more will reach the colon, along with dietary fibre.

In the large intestine

Hundreds of different species of bacteria live in the large intestine. Many of them break down various types of dietary fibre and any carbohydrates which have escaped digestion in the small intestine. During this bacterial digestion (also known as 'fermentation'), more kilojoules of energy are made available. Most dietary fibre is broken down by these helpful bacteria but some types of fibre, such as lignin, are not changed at all and are eventually excreted. The bacteria themselves multiply by the million as they ferment fibre and carbohydrates and they later contribute bulk to the faecal material which is excreted. The more bacteria present, the greater the quantity of faeces excreted.

The fermentation of fibre and carbohydrate by bacteria produces large quantities of gas. The more fibre and complex carbohydrate eaten, the more bacteria and the larger the volume of gas produced. Fibre holds water so a high fibre diet also leads to larger volumes of faeces as well as a greater production of valuable organic acids. Eating more fibre helps prevent the small hard faeces which occur in constipation.

About 1.5 kg of food residues and water enter the large intestine each day. The contents move slowly through the large intestine and total transit time from the caecum (the first part of the large intestine) to the rectum varies greatly. Australian studies show transit times ranging from 24 to 36 hours. Men usually have faster transit times than women. Some people have extremely slow transit times. Studies in the United Kingdom have shown that about 5% of men and 11% of women have transit times of more than 120 hours. This may be influenced by the typical low intake of dietary fibre in the United Kingdom. Older people, women and those who have low fibre diets have the longest transit time.

During the passage of food residues through the large intestine, a large amount of water is reabsorbed and faeces change from liquid to a more solid consistency. Approximately 100-150g of faeces are passed each day. If water is not reabsorbed because the passage is too rapid, diarrhoea results. If transit time is too slow, more water is reabsorbed and faeces become hard and pellet-like. The passage of food residues is controlled by muscular contractions of the bowel wall. The slower transit time and smaller faeces in women occur partly because more water has been absorbed from their faeces.

> Better to burp and bear the shame
> Than squelch the belch and bear the pain. Anonymous.

Why do we produce gas?

Gas is an essential and unavoidable part of the normal process of digesting food.

Some gas in the intestine, particularly in the stomach, but also in the colon, comes from swallowed air. Most of the gas we pass is produced in the colon by bacteria as they break down some kinds of complex carbohydrate and most types of dietary fibre. These good and useful bacteria grow and multiply by using the gases produced as a source of energy for themselves.

The bacteria also break down old cells which have been shed from the lining of the gastrointestinal tract. Even if you were fasting, you still produce gas from this source.

Producing gas is usually a sign of a good high fibre diet and of good health. It is not abnormal and any inconvenience it may cause is social not medical.

The sulphur compounds that cause gas after eating cabbage double between the 5th and 7th minute of cooking. To reduce gas after eating cabbage, cook it for less than 5 minutes.

Where does gas come from?

Some gas comes from air which we swallow, or, more correctly, suck in. We swallow air when we eat and drink and also at other times. This air must get out. Some of it is released by burping or belching.

Most of the oxygen from the air we swallow is absorbed from the stomach and duodenum (the first part of the small intestine). Beyond the small intestine, there is no oxygen—the environment in the colon is anaerobic (meaning 'without oxygen'). Most of the bacteria in the colon can only survive in anaerobic conditions.

Some of the nitrogen from the swallowed air is also absorbed from the upper parts of the intestine but some passes to the colon, ultimately to be passed as flatus.

Most of the gas passed from the anus is generated within the intestinal tract. It is composed of **carbon dioxide, hydrogen, methane, nitrogen and sulphur dioxide**. Apart from sulphur dioxide, the gases we pass are odourless. However, some other volatile substances excreted with these gases may contribute an odour.

Carbon dioxide gas comes from the interaction between stomach acid and alkaline secretions of the small intestine and also from fermentation of fibre and carbohydrate in the colon. Some carbon dioxide also diffuses into the colon from the bloodstream, especially at high altitudes.

Hydrogen is produced when bacteria in the large bowel (the colon) ferment dietary fibre, some starches or certain types of sugars. Hydrogen can be used by bacteria or converted by them to **methane** or **sulphur dioxide**.

Nitrogen comes mainly from air we breathe in or swallow.

Most of the foods we eat are digested in the small intestine and their nutrients are absorbed from there. However, dietary fibre and some types of starches and sugars are not digested by the enzymes in the small intestine. Instead, bacteria that live in the large bowel ferment them. In the process, the bacteria produce fatty acids which nourish and protect the cells lining the bowel and help prevent bowel cancer.

The fermentation also produces gases, some of which the bacteria use as an energy supply to help them survive and multiply. The rest of the gas is absorbed into the blood and eventually leaves the body in the breath, or it is passed through the anus as flatus.

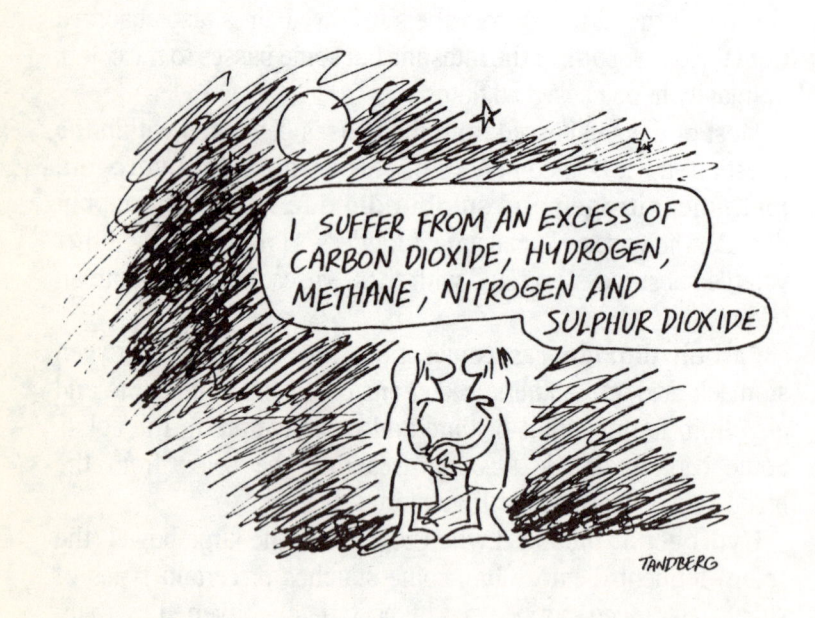

Does everyone produce gas?

Yes. People of all ages and both sexes produce gas every day.

Babies begin to produce gas a few days after birth when bacteria start to grow in the bowel. Babies also swallow air when sucking. Some of this is burped and some passes through to the colon.

Children produce a different mixture of gases from adults. They do not usually produce much methane gas until they reach their teens. Breast-fed babies do not produce any methane. No one yet knows why this is so, but children may not have the same bacteria as adults. However, as they grow up, children tend to develop the same type of bacteria as their parents.

St Augustine believed that once man disobeyed God, he was unable to obey himself. He therefore considered that any involuntary bodily functions, including flatulence, signalled man's fall from grace.

How much gas is normal?

The amount of gas you make depends partly on your diet and partly on the kind of bacteria that live in your bowel. The average person produces 400-2400 mL of gas a day, usually passed in portions of 30-120 mL. If you imagine a party balloon, half blown up, you will have some idea of the volume of the average production of 1500 mL of gas.

At any one time, most people will have 150-200 mL of gas in the gastrointestinal tract. The process of producing gas, and its use by bacteria and passage as flatus, is continuous.

The number of times someone passes gas varies. One study done many years ago on young men found that the average number of emissions in 24 hours was 10-15. Our own study, just completed, using many more people of different ages and both sexes found the daily average among women was 7 emissions and among men was 12. There was a large variation, ranging from 3 to 38. Gas production depended partly on the amount of dietary fibre consumed. At low fibre intakes, there was less gas. Those on a high fibre diet had more frequent emissions. However, some people who consumed little fibre produced a lot of gas, while a few who ate a lot of fibre did not pass gas very much.

Some people pass small volumes of gas often and others pass larger volumes less often. How often you fart depends on the sensitivity of the walls of your rectum. If your rectum is sensitive to a small amount of distension, you will pass small volumes more often than if your rectum tolerates greater distension.

When should we regard gas as excessive?

It is difficult to define 'excessive gas'. What some people regard as normal is seen by others as excessive. It is usually other people, such as spouses, workmates or children, who complain about problems of gas in those they live and work with.

Adults complain more about the volume of gas they produce than children. This may be either because they feel they 'blow up' or 'bloat' more or because adults produce and pass more gas.

When many people complain about excess gas, it is not the volume that concerns them but the smell and the fear that they will not be able to control it.

Those with 'bloating' or irritable bowel syndrome (see page 35) produce similar quantities of gas to everyone else but their sensitivity to the same volume of gas is greater.

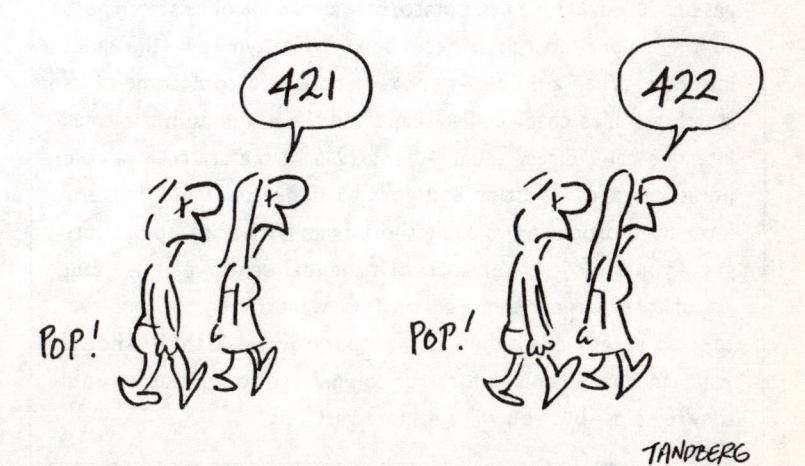

Is gas a greater problem in older people?

As we grow older, we do not produce more gas, but the bowel becomes less elastic and more sensitive to being distended by the usual volume of gas produced. Many elderly people are less able to hold gas in their rectum and so pass wind more frequently. This may be due to weaker pelvic muscles which control the process of holding and passing gas.

Previous pregnancies or surgery may weaken the pelvic muscles and make it more difficult to control passing of gas. Some elderly people may therefore expel gas at times when it is less socially acceptable to do so.

Eating a potato hot, cold or reheated may change the amount of gas it causes. The more starch that gets through to the colon, the more gas produced. With a hot potato, only about 3% of its starch goes to the colon; most is broken down by enzymes in the small intestine. When a potato is cooked and left to cool, some of its starch granules change their shape and the enzymes in the small intestine can't digest them. About 12% of the starch in a cold potato escapes digestion and goes to the colon where bacteria ferment it, producing valuable short chain fatty acids - plus more gas. If you cook your potato, cool it and then reheat it later, about 7% of its starch goes to the colon. If you want to increase your level of social acceptability, then eat your potatoes while they're hot. If you want more benefits for your colon, leave your potatoes until they're cold—but you will get more gas!

When do we produce most gas?

Some people produce more gas in the morning, others produce more in the evening. Almost everyone produces more after meals and less while sleeping. Gas production generally increases about an hour after meals. A large meal usually produces more gas than a small meal. Those troubled by gas may find it better to eat 'small and often' rather than having three main meals a day.

During the night when we are asleep, muscular movements in the colon slow down. If you pass gas early in the morning, it will be mainly nitrogen. Early morning gases contain little hydrogen or carbon dioxide because these will have been absorbed into the blood and expired on the breath during the night.

If you are tense or anxious, you may have more gas. Some comes from swallowing more air and some is extra hydrogen which is produced and trapped in the right side of the colon. The reason why feeling tense has this effect is unknown.

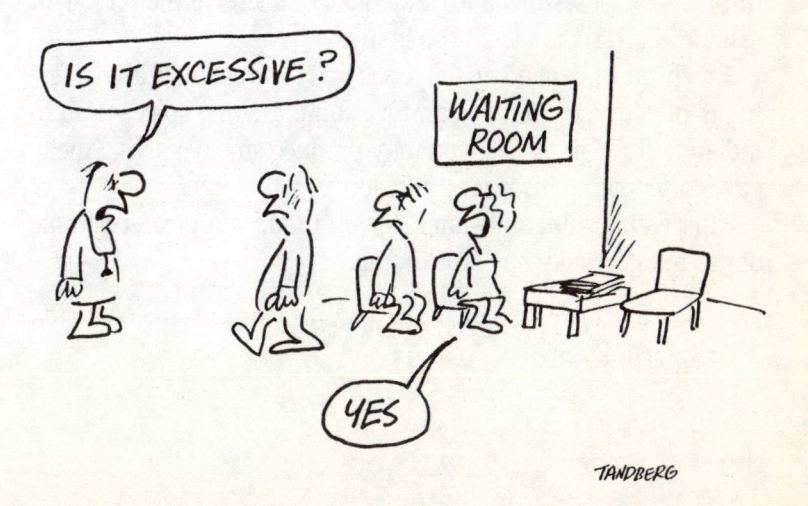

Does gas production depend on what you have just eaten or on what you ate the day before?

Gases are being produced in the colon continuously, especially if you eat foods high in dietary fibre and certain starches. Gases in the stomach usually come from swallowed air and will be most apparent soon after eating or drinking.

Some people complain of gas within a few minutes of eating; others an hour or so later. It normally takes about an hour and a half for some of the food from a meal to pass from the stomach, through the small intestine and into the colon where fermentation begins. If the meal was high in protein and fat, it takes much longer until the entire meal has cleared the stomach and small intestine. The first part of a meal will get to the colon quickly and as soon as it comes into contact with the millions of bacteria there, some gas is produced. This process then continues for many hours. For most people, the length of time food takes to pass through the intestine and undergo complete fermentation of residues in the colon is 24–36 hours.

Smelly gases depend on the foods you have eaten. Within a few hours of eating certain spices, for example, some spices used in Indian and Asian dishes, you may produce smelly gases. Smelly gases after eating meat may take longer to emerge.

After eating fibre and starches, you produce a greater volume of gas but it usually has little aroma.

How can you produce gas within minutes of finishing a meal?

Flatus within a few minutes of eating is due to a reflex reaction from the stomach causing residues from the previous meal to squeeze into the colon from the last section of the small intestine. The change in the contents of the colon and the movement of the muscular walls increases the pressure so some gas is expelled.

After meals, the muscular movements of the walls of the colon increase. The movement may increase gas by mixing fibre and any carbohydrate not digested in the small intestine with bacteria. These muscular movements also propel gas onwards through the colon towards the anus.

Choose your onions carefully!

Different types of onions reportedly produce different amounts of gas. 90g of Dutch onions produced 58 mL/hour; 105 g of Egyptian onions produced 101 mL/hour; 115 g Italian onions produced 181 mL/hour. For the chemists, the active component in onions seems to be gamma-glutamyl-S-alkyl cysteine. For the non-chemists, that's a sulphur compound which is converted to methylmercaptan - another sulphur compound with a potent sulphurous aroma. Onions, garlic and leeks also contain fructans, polymers of the sugar fructose. These also produce gas.

Do men and women produce the same amount of gas?

As you can imagine, it is not easy to measure the volumes of gas produced. Some limited research suggested that both sexes produced similar volumes of gas. However, the volume does vary with the amount and type of food eaten so anyone of either sex who eats more foods high in fibre and starch will produce more gas. Our own study found that men passed gas more often than women.

Some types of bacteria in the colon convert a large volume of hydrogen to a smaller volume of methane. This uses up more of the volume of gas, leaving less to be passed. More women than men have these bacteria and those who have them may pass less gas.

Women generally have a slower transit of contents through the intestinal tract. They also form smaller stools which are more alkaline. These factors may favour the growth of methane-producing bacteria. We still don't fully understand why women are different in this respect but it could be due to an interaction between the many gut hormones and female reproductive hormones. Any possible benefits or disadvantages are also not yet understood.

In our study, women had fewer emissions of gas then men, but the variation in gas in both men and women covered a wide range. The range for men was 3–38 emissions a day; for women it was 3–32. Women said that gas had an odour less than half the time; men reported an odour more than two-thirds of the time.

Do women on hormone replacement therapy produce more gas?

Many women on hormone replacement therapy (HRT) report that they produce more gas. This is due to the progestogen component of HRT which slows the activity of muscles in the intestine, producing constipation, distension and increased gas. The smaller the dose of progestogen in HRT, the fewer the side effects. The extra gas is not medically harmful, only socially embarrassing.

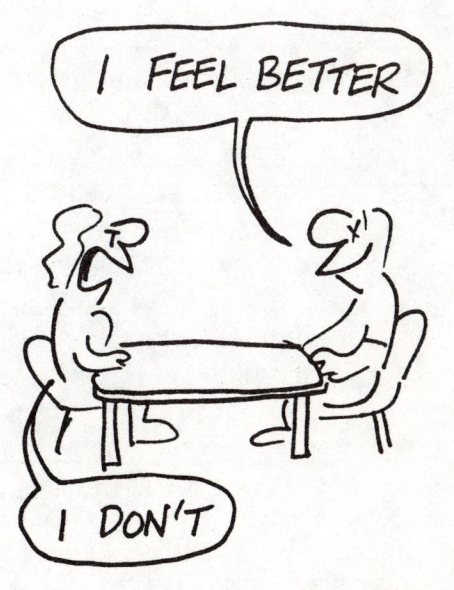

Can gases from humans affect the environment in the same way gases from cows can?

Both carbon dioxide and methane are greenhouse gases. Human methane adds to the methane produced by animals. Scientists are concerned that an increase in greenhouse gases will raise the temperature of the earth. However, humans produce much less methane than animals and it remains to be seen if we are a threat to our own future. An average weight cow produces 250 litres of methane a day.

> 'The hungry sheep look up, and are not fed,
> But, swoln with wind and the rank mist they draw,
> Rot inwardly and foul contagion spread'. John Milton.

Why does gas sometimes make a noise when it is being passed and sometimes the process is quiet?

Cultural constraints have a major influence on noise. In most societies, audible flatus is not socially acceptable. In general, there is more noise from a larger volume of gas. The 'pitch' depends on the diameter of the anal canal. A narrow opening produces a higher 'pitch' than a relaxed anus. Sitting, especially on a toilet, tends to produce a louder noise than standing. Haemorrhoids do not alter the pitch or intensity of the sound.

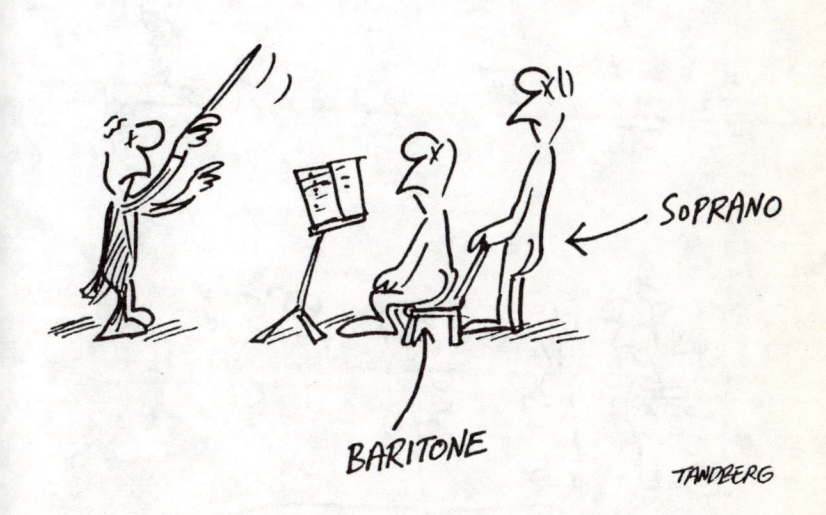

Is it harmful to hold on to gas?

It is not harmful to hold on to gas but it can become a habit which makes you feel bloated and uncomfortable because the lower bowel is blown up like a balloon. It may cause pain.

Pain in the bowel is usually due to distension. This is not surprising as the bowel has many sensitive nerves passing through its walls. When you pass gas, the pain disappears.

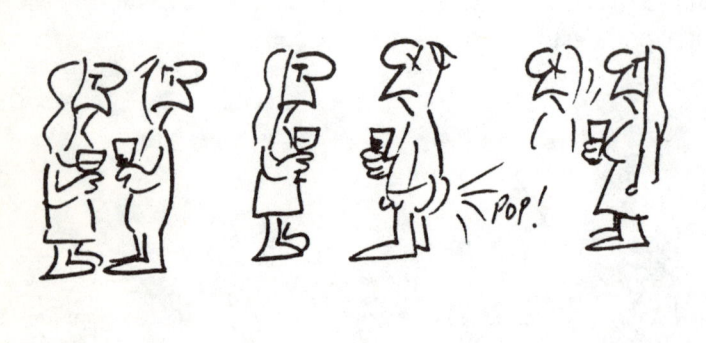

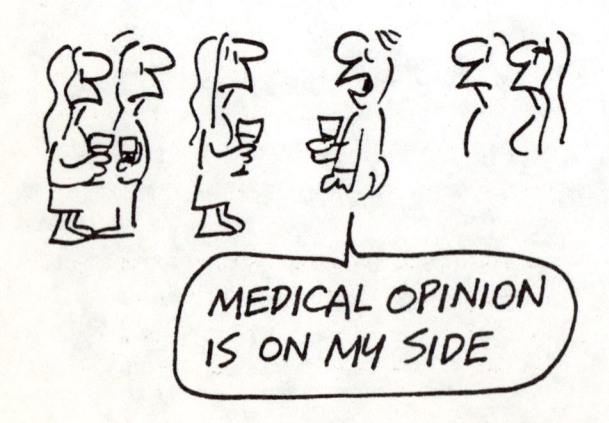

Why do gases produced in the colon escape from the anus rather than coming out of the mouth?

It is true that gases usually bubble to the top, but there is a valve at the junction of the small intestine and the colon which prevents fluids and gas passing back into the small intestine. This valve has a similar effect to the valve at the junction of the oesophagus and the stomach which stops acid from the stomach refluxing into the oesophagus.

The muscular contractions of the bowel also propel the contents towards the rectum.

Aiming for the *Guinness Book of Records?*
One man, who used the pseudonym L.O Sutalf, passed an average of 34 emissions of flatus a day. Adding a litre of milk to his diet, he increased this to 90. When he drank nothing but milk for two days, he farted 141 times in 24 hours, including 70 in one four-hour period! The man had problems with lactose! When he stopped using milk, he reduced his daily flatus total to 25 emissions. By careful testing of different foods, he eventually worked out that he needed a diet without milk, onions, beans, celery, carrot, raisins, bananas, apricots, prune juice, pretzels, bagels, wheatgerm, Brussels sprouts, pastries, potatoes, eggplant, apples, citrus fruits and bread to reduce his daily total to 19 or less. Fortunately, not everyone has his problems and not everyone would find his diet beneficial.

How does the body distinguish between the urge to pass faeces or flatus?

The lining of the anal canal has a profuse supply of exquisitely sensitive nerves that can distinguish between a light touch, pain, heat and cold. These nerves can also distinguish between faecal matter and gas.

The muscular area of the anus over which we have voluntary control (called the 'anal sphincter) preserves anal continence. When the rectum is empty, the sphincter lengthens, but when the rectum contains faeces or gas, the sphincter zone shortens and brings the contents of the rectum into contact with the highly sensitive part of the anal canal. The sensations in the anal canal then give a fine level of control to anal continence.

The rectum is sensitive to a volume of contents as little as 10 mL. As the volume of the contents increases, it reaches a particular pressure (which may vary between individuals) and triggers the rectum to empty. This reaction can be controlled by social training and changes in daily routine can alter the emptying response. Many people find that when they are away from their regular toilet, they do not get their usual urge to defaecate.

When rectal pressure increases rapidly, there is an urgent sense to empty the rectum. This may occur with a sudden increase in gas or from watery faeces in diarrhoea.

> 'He o hitte shiri tsubome' (translates as *No use scrunching your buttocks after a fart*). Japanese proverb.

What gases do we produce?

When bacteria ferment starches, sugars and dietary fibre in the colon, carbon dioxide and hydrogen are produced. **Hydrogen** is the major gas produced, most of it in the right side of the colon. About two-thirds of the 12 litres of hydrogen we produce each day is absorbed from the colon into the blood and is carried to the lungs. We breathe it out in expired air.

Some of the hydrogen is converted by special bacteria to **methane**, an odourless gas.

To produce one molecule of methane, the methane-producing bacteria use four molecules of hydrogen and one of carbon dioxide. This gets rid of a lot of hydrogen. Most people have some methane-producing bacteria but only about half the population have significant numbers of them.

More women than men produce methane. About 60% of women but only about 40% of men make significant quantities of this gas. Children under the age of 4 or 5 don't usually produce it at all. Because methane uses up more hydrogen, it is likely that anyone with with methane-producing bacteria will produce less gas than someone without these bacteria.

Another type of bacteria use hydrogen to make **hydrogen sulphide** (a smelly gas with an aroma of rotten eggs) and other sulphur compounds. The methane-producing and the sulphate-reducing bacteria compete with each other to use the hydrogen. Not everyone has significant numbers of both these types of bacteria. Most people have either a dominant colony of bacteria that produce methane or they have bacteria that use sulphate to produce sulphides.

If you are one of the people with bacteria which change sulphates, your bacteria may dominate the methane-producing type and win the competition for hydrogen, using it up before the methane-producing bacteria can get it.

The processes of making methane and hydrogen sulphide reduce the volume of hydrogen gas in the colon. Any hydrogen not used by the bacteria is excreted on the breath or is passed through the anus.

The bacteria which produce methane are present mainly in the left colon. Those that produce hydrogen sulphide gas and sulphur compounds are found throughout the colon. They increase if you have a diet containing lots of sulphur.

Most of the sulphur we consume in the diet is absorbed from the small intestine. However, if you eat a lot of sulphur-containing foods, some will get through to the colon. As the bacteria use the sulphur, they multiply and may overwhelm any methane-producing bacteria.

Sulphur comes naturally from the loss of old cells throughout the intestine. It also comes from sulphur-containing amino acids (part of proteins in foods) or from sulphur compounds in vegetables, especially garlic, onion and cabbage. A lot of sulphur comes from sodium metabisulphite added to foods and beverages as a preservative and from other sulphur-containing food additives. Most breads, beer, wine (especially white wines and cask wines), cider, dried fruits, orange or apple juices made from concentrate or with added preservative, and potato crisps and chips contain these sulphur compounds.

Another type of bacteria may use **carbon dioxide** and hydrogen to produce acetic acid. There is not much of this acid produced and most carbon dioxide is reabsorbed and expired in the breath.

Some other gases can make up about a third of the gases passed. Most of this gas is probably **nitrogen**. Some of it comes from swallowed air, some may come from gas which has diffused from the blood into the bowel and some may have come from the amino acids that make up protein in the diet.

Ammonia can also be produced in the colon from amino acids and other components of protein. Ammonia is a toxic gas but if there are plenty of bacteria (for example, from a high fibre diet), they will use up this ammonia. This is a reason why keeping proteins and carbohydrates separate (as in Food Combining theories) is wrong. Anyone who eats a lot of protein foods should also eat high fibre foods such as potatoes, cereals, grains, bread or beans.

Joseph Pujol was born in Marseilles in 1857. He delighted music hall audiences at the Moulin Rouge in Paris during the 1890s with his musical performances - with a difference. Pujol, stage-named 'le Petomane' (the Fartomaniac), had mastered the art of taking in air through his anus and expelling it at will. His repertoire included bird sounds, tremulos reminiscent of violins, a solo falsetto, a 10-second aria mimicking tearing calico, a rendition of Au Clair de la Lune and blowing out a candle from a distance of just under half a metre. His act was a sensation and audiences rolled in the aisles at his antics. He was eventually replaced by a substitute 'femme-petomane' but had the last word when he uncovered concealed bellows under her skirts.

Is it good or bad to produce methane gas?

There were some reports a few years ago that methane producers had a higher incidence of bowel cancer. More recent research has not confirmed this.

A higher percentage of those with diverticular disease produce methane. This is probably related to the slow transit time which usually occurs in this condition. (Diverticula occur when muscular contractions increase pressure in the colon and cause small pockets to form in weak spots in the wall of the colon. They are more common in those who have a low fibre diet and small hard faeces. A high fibre diet produces bulkier, softer faeces.) When food residues take longer to pass through the intestine, any methane-producing bacteria present will multiply.

Few people with Crohn's disease of the colon (a condition in which various areas of the intestine become inflamed) produce methane while a higher than normal percentage of people with cystic fibrosis are methane-producers.

More research is needed to uncover the relevance of methane and solve the mystery of why some healthy people produce methane and others produce very little.

'Ill blows the wind that profits nobody'. *Henry VI*, William Shakespeare.

Are some gases produced faster than others?

Some sugars pass quickly through the stomach to the small intestine. If they are not digested there, they will pass rapidly to the large bowel. They are fermented quickly in the right side of the colon, producing hydrogen gas in the process. Some of the hydrogen is excreted on the breath and some passes from the anus.

Oligosaccharides (made up of several sugar molecules joined together) may also be fermented quickly by bacteria and produce a lot of gas. Most seeds and beans are rich in the oligosaccharides called raffinose, verbascose and stachyose. These are responsible for much of the high gas production after eating beans.

When carbohydrates are more complex, for example, some of the starches from breads, grains, cereals or potatoes, they usually take longer to ferment. Valuable short chain fatty acids are produced during this fermentation of carbohydrate. Most of the action takes place in the right side of the colon. The bacteria are of two major types: one type changes hydrogen to methane; another converts it to hydrogen sulphide. Both types of bacteria are very efficient in using up the hydrogen produced in the right colon. They may use up all the hydrogen in this process so there is none left to pass as flatus.

Is there any way to produce less gas?

If you are producing an excessive amount of gas because you are lactose-intolerant (see page 45), avoiding milk and ice cream will help relieve gas and any bloating or discomfort associated with it. You will need to find alternative sources of calcium, such as cheese, fortified soya milk (which may also cause gas) or a calcium supplement. If you are not lactose-intolerant, removing milk from your diet will have no effect on gas.

You may produce less gas if you eat less dietary fibre but fibre is important for good health. Gases produced from dietary fibre are a social inconvenience but a medical advantage, especially to keep the bowel healthy.

There are therapies for excessive gas. Before considering these, remember that what you think is excessive may be quite normal.

Many people ask for antibiotics, expecting they will destroy bacteria and therefore reduce gas. In fact, gas production may *increase* with antibiotics, possibly because antibiotics reduce the bacteria which normally use up hydrogen gas and convert it into methane or sulphur compounds. Some antibiotics can also cause a form of colitis.

Tablets sold as Degas, No-gas or Phazyme contain a substance called simethicone which can reduce surface tension in the colon and cause gas bubbles to join together. This makes burping easier and may also reduce flatus. These tablets have no adverse side effects and are often an effective treatment.

Anticholinergic drugs such as Colofac block nerves that stimulate muscular activity in the gastrointestinal tract. They reduce pressure in the colon and ease pain but have no effect on the amount of gas produced.

Activated charcoal has an extensive surface area and has been shown to reduce gas after eating beans. It may be worth a try. Charcoal is an odourless, tasteless product made by burning wood pulp. It is 'activated' by using an oxidising gas at high temperatures. It is used in military gas masks and is given after someone has inadvertently consumed certain poisons, including some drugs.

The main *treatment* for gas is to recognise that the amount you produce may not be abnormal. If you burp a lot, it is probably because you swallow a lot of air when eating or drinking, without realising it, perhaps because you are tense. If you are concerned that you produce a lot more than the average quantity of flatus, or if you have any pain, diarrhoea or constipation associated with gas, see your doctor. If tests for lactose intolerance are positive, cutting back on milk and ice cream will help reduce the amount of gas produced. If tests for lactose intolerance are negative, there is no point in avoiding milk. If you want to reduce gas production, you may need to avoid beans and foods such as some spices and some vegetables.

Jerusalem artichokes score zero in the aphrodisiac stakes. They have a particularly high level of inulin, a polysaccharide which cannot be digested. It ferments in the colon, producing copious quantities of gas.

Why do you produce more gas in an aeroplane?

Gravitational pull, vibration and stress can increase gas production. The volume of a gas also increases as the pressure around it decreases. Flying in an unpressurised plane would therefore cause intestinal gases to expand, causing abdominal distension and pain.

Mountaineers, astronauts and cosmonauts produce gas which is rich in carbon dioxide (more than 75% of the total gases produced). This comes from carbon dioxide diffusing from their tissues and blood into the colon. At normal altitudes, very little such diffusion occurs.

Mountain climbers at an altitude of 10,500 metres produce gas that is 80% carbon dioxide, most of which diffuses from the blood into the colon (the opposite to the normal movement of this gas). Astronauts have the same problem.

Why do scuba divers sometimes suffer with excess gas?

There are several reasons why scuba divers sometimes get excess gas in the gut. Inexperienced scuba divers tend to swallow more air. During their descent, if they forcefully breath out while holding the nose and keeping the lips tightly closed, air can be forced into the stomach.

Drinking carbonated beverages, eating beans or having a fatty meal soon before diving also increases air in the stomach.

During the ascent from the dive, gases in the intestine expand as the surrounding atmospheric pressure decreases. This may cause abdominal distension and a colicky pain.

Treatment is for divers to slow the rate at which they come up from a dive or wait until they pass some gas from the colon. Occasionally, the diver may need to go down to a higher pressure and come up again more slowly. Recompression is rarely needed.

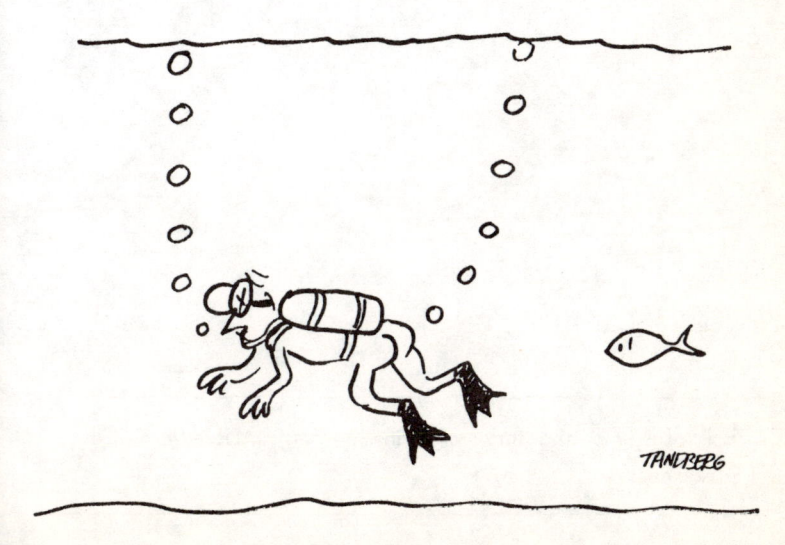

Can gases explode in the bowel?

Boys (we are not being sexist, but we know of no instances in girls) often delight in seeing if the flatus emerging from their mates can be lit with a match. If the 'mate' is a producer of methane gas, the match will flare! Hydrogen gas will also ignite.

Explosions can occur within the colon if an electric current used during surgery ignites hydrogen or methane gases. Flatus can easily contain a great enough concentration of these gases for the schoolboy pranks mentioned above. In practice, before examining the colon for bowel cancer or to remove polyps using a colonoscope, the bowel is cleaned out and the concentration of any gases will be too low for there to be any danger of an explosion occurring.

'Full of sound and fury, signifying nothing'. *Macbeth*, William Shakespeare.

Do mood and emotions affect gas?

Changes in mood, especially tension—either acute or chronic—can increase the amount of gas in the large bowel in at least three ways.

The increase in gas may occur because food passes more rapidly through the small intestine without enough time to be digested in the normal manner. Bacteria in the large bowel then ferment the food, producing more hydrogen gas in the process. For some reason which is not known, this hydrogen is not converted to methane, which would reduce its volume.

Tension may also increase the amount of gas being held in the bowel, particularly in the right side of the colon where there are few bacteria that either produce methane or reduce sulphate.

When you are tense, you are also more likely to swallow air and this will increase the amount of nitrogen in the bowel.

Changes in mood do not affect the amount of methane produced.

Do people with gall stones produce more gas?

Burping and bloating are more common in people with gall stones and they often improve after the gall bladder is removed. However, gas is not responsible for the pain of gall stones and you do not cure flatulence by removing the gall bladder.

> 'Quando il malato scoppia, il medico piange!' (translates as *When the sick man farts, the doctor cries*). Old saying from Southern Italy, akin to our saying 'an apple a day keeps the doctor away'.

Is irritable bowel syndrome caused by gas?

Irritable bowel syndrome is one of the most common gastrointestinal complaints. It affects people of all ages and both sexes and is characterised by pain, diarrhoea, or more commonly, constipation and bloating or distension. The pain is usually better after passing flatus or after a bowel motion, both of which reduce pressure in the colon.

Many people with irritable bowel complain of excessive gas. In fact, tests to measure gas volume by flushing all gases out with an inert gas such as argon show that people with irritable bowel syndrome don't produce any more gas than other people. However, this condition makes people more sensitive to and have more pain from the pressure of a normal volume of gas. They may have some disorder of the muscles of the bowel wall which interferes with the normal passage of gas through the intestine.

Why do you get more gas if you have a hiatus hernia?

A hiatus hernia occurs when a little bit of the stomach bulges upwards through the diaphragm. There is a valve at the lower end of the oesophagus which normally controls movement of food into the stomach and stops food and stomach contents refluxing back into the oesophagus. A hiatus hernia weakens this valve and allows stomach acid and gas to reflux, causing heartburn and burping. After an operation to fix the hiatus hernia, it can be impossible to burp and excess gas in the stomach can then cause great discomfort. Medication can reduce the amount of stomach acid produced and relieve the burping associated with hiatus hernia.

When you burp, you swallow or suck more air into the stomach than is burped out. Some of this extra air passes through the gastrointestinal tract to the colon and eventually emerges as flatus.

Why do you get more wind after an operation?

After abdominal surgery, muscular contractions of the gastrointestinal tract may stop for a few days. Gas continues to accumulate, but with fewer muscular contractions, it is not passed as flatus. The gas causes distension and the distension causes abdominal pain. As the bowel muscles begin to work again, gas is passed and the pain disappears.

> 'The intestines are the home of tempests: in them is formed gas, as in the clouds'. Brillat-Savarin.

Do some foods produce more gas than others?

Foods high in dietary fibre cause gas and the more fibre you eat, the more likely you are to produce more gas. There are also other compounds in foods that cause gas. For example, cabbage, cauliflower, broccoli, Brussels sprouts, turnips, dried beans and seeds (fennel, sunflower, poppy) contain substances which lead to a high production of gases. Onions, garlic and leeks produce gas in many people and different types of onions may have a more potent effect in some people. Beans are notorious for producing lots of gas (see page 40).

Different people produce different amounts of gas after eating similar amounts of the same type of food. Some people have different perceptions of the amount of gas they produce and what one person regards as a lot is seen as quite normal by someone else. There are also genuine differences between individuals. A food which does not cause gas in one person may generate it in another. You are not abnormal just because you produce more gas than someone else after eating a particular food. This is simply one of nature's many variations.

However, if you produce much more gas than the average 7-12 emissions a day, you may either be swallowing a lot of air when you eat and drink, or something you are eating is fermenting excessively in your colon. The most common culprit is lactose from milk (see page 45). Lactose is in all milks. Some modified low fat milks, where the low fat component of the milk has been concentrated to give higher calcium levels and more 'body', have higher quantities of lactose. Cheese contains almost no lactose and is not a problem.

Is there any way to eat a high fibre diet without producing a lot of gas?

No, it is neither possible nor desirable to stop gas production. However, if you increase fibre intake gradually you will have fewer problems with gas than if you suddenly adopt a high fibre diet. The benefits of dietary fibre far outweigh the social inconvenience of producing gas. The bacteria which use the gas from fibre also produce valuable substances called short chain fatty acids which keep the cells of the walls of the colon healthy. They may also help prevent bowel cancer.

People who eat more dietary fibre and starch usually produce large stools. There is now good evidence that those who produce larger stools are less likely to develop bowel cancer.

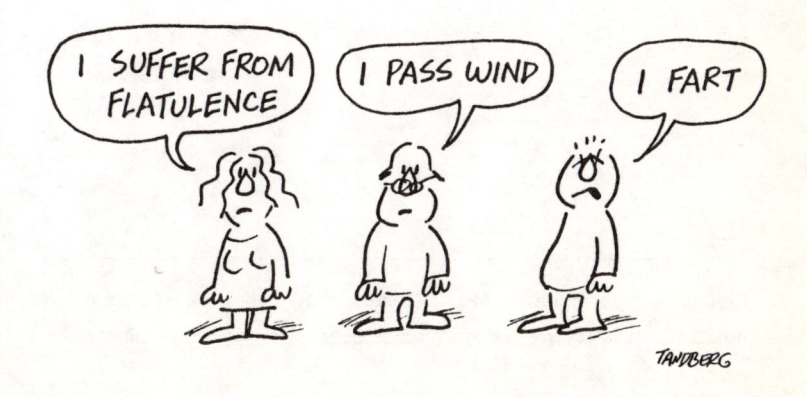

Why do beans cause so much gas?

Beans are one of the highest sources of valuable types of fibre. When this fibre is fermented by bacteria in the colon, it will increase gas. Beans also contain some complex sugars called oligosaccharides. These are not digested in the small intestine but are fermented by bacteria in the colon and produce larger quantities of gases, especially carbon dioxide. Soya beans are usually considered to be the greatest source of gas.

For those who like such details, soya beans' oligosaccharides are mainly raffinose and stachyose with smaller amounts of pinitol, galactopinitol and manninotriose. Other beans and peas contain larger amounts of an oligosaccharide called verbascose. Humans do not have the enzymes in the small intestine to digest any of these substances but the bacteria in the colon do.

If the oligosaccharides are removed or soaked out of beans, they still cause some gas, probably because they have so much dietary fibre.

Mediterranean folklore has it that adding half a teaspoon of mustard seeds to the water in which beans are cooked eliminates much of the gas.

How can I decrease the amount of gas from beans?

There are several ways to decrease gas from legumes (dried beans and peas).

Introduce beans gradually into your diet so bacteria in the bowel do not multiply suddenly. Although a gradual introduction of beans doesn't reduce the *amount* of gas produced, it allows your bowel to develop tolerance so you experience less physical discomfort.

Soak beans overnight and pour away the soaking water. Some of the offending oligosaccharides will have dissolved into the water. After soaking for 18 hours, 90% of the oligosaccharides disappear from black-eyed beans, 88% from pink beans, 30–51% of those in cannellini, kidney and pinto beans and between 45 and 80% from the tiny Indian black gram beans.

If you eat the clear-looking skin on dried beans and peas, you may reduce gas production because the skin contains some minerals, including manganese, which can bind some substances needed for gases to form.

Try adding about half a teaspoon of mustard seeds to the water when cooking beans. Some cooks in Mediterranean countries are convinced it works. It's worth a try and seems to have some effect. Some studies have also shown that certain spices prevent some bacteria from producing gases.

Sprouting beans may reduce their oligosaccharides and so reduce gas. In some cases, sprouting has little effect on the flatus caused by beans. This is probably because some of the oligosaccharides, especially raffinose, are used during the germination but other oligosaccharides are formed by the germinating seed.

Soya beans can be cooked and fermented by adding a species *Rhizopus* bacteria to produce tempeh. Tempeh does not cause excessive intestinal gas partly because the oligosaccharides are used by the bacteria during the fermentation and partly because the fermented tempeh contains an antibiotic substance which acts against gas-forming organisms in the colon.

Idli, a fermented mixture of black gram and rice, produces much less gas than the black gram beans alone. During the fermentation, the verbascose in the beans is used up and so does not ferment in the colon. Other beans fermented with rice show similar reductions in gas.

Eating soya beans in the form of tofu also helps reduce gas, although it also deprives the body of the dietary fibre of the soya bean. Tofu is made by treating soya bean milk with calcium or magnesium salts so that the curd precipitates. This is then partially dried to form tofu. It does not cause extra gas. Some types of soya bean milk, however, may produce gas as they still contain raffinose and stachyose—oligosaccharides which are fermented in the colon.

Most of the complex sugars responsible for gases produced after eating beans accumulate in mature-age beans. Green immature beans cause much less flatulence.

Is there any way to stop cabbage and cauliflower causing gas?

Cabbage and other related vegetables such as Brussels sprouts, cauliflower, broccoli and turnips, contain several potent sulphur compounds, including hydrogen sulphide, methyl sulphide and mercaptans. These react together to form compounds called trisulphides. The longer you cook the vegetables, the more of these trisulphides form, the stronger the flavour and smell, and the more gas they will cause. The hydrogen sulphide in cabbage also increases with the length of time the cabbage is cooked. If you want less gas after eating cabbage, the trick is to cook it briefly. Try stir-frying it rather than boiling or steaming.

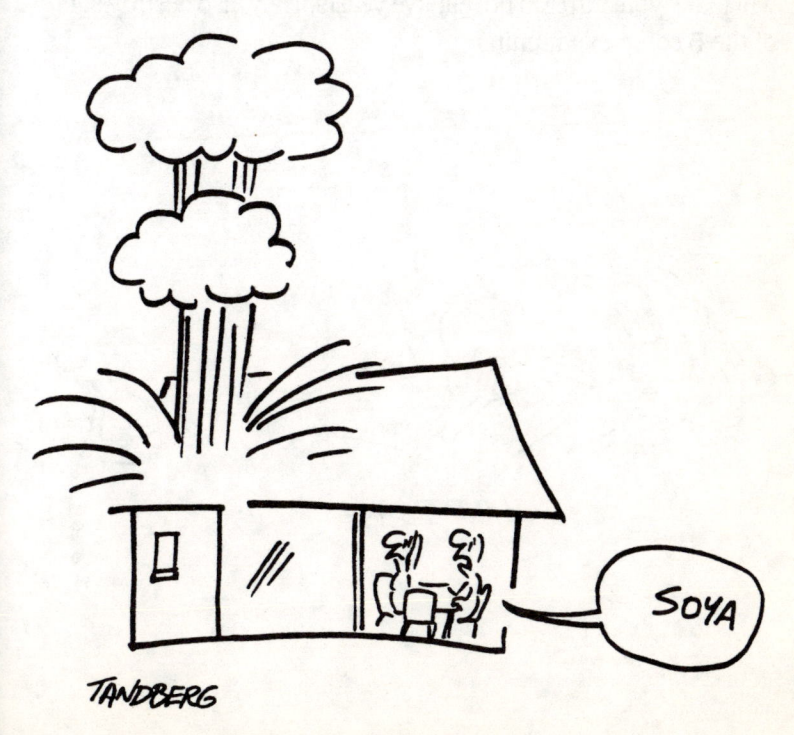

Do yeasts in foods cause gas?

Yeast or candida in the bowel does not cause gas. Some people recommend a special diet which includes restrictions on sugar, bread and some fruits to treat candidiasis. With such a diet, there may be less gas as there is less carbohydrate in the diet, and therefore, less carbohydrate will reach the colon for fermentation. Yeasts are sometimes found in the colon but their ability to make gas does not compare with that of the other bacteria present. A yeast-free diet doesn't always get rid of the yeasts. There are also many people with yeasts in their colon but no symptoms.

Eating live yeasts, for example, baker's yeast or by eating uncooked bread dough produces a lot of gas in the stomach which will make you burp. Do not eat live yeasts. They also destroy some of the B complex vitamins.

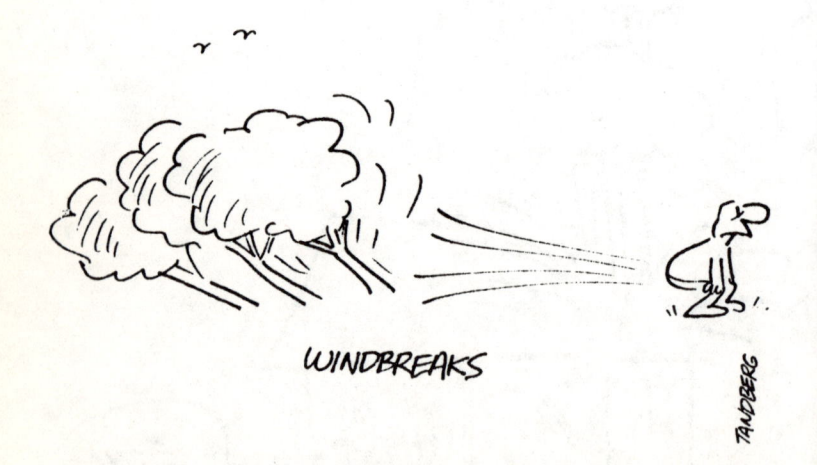

WINDBREAKS

Do dairy products increase gas?

Milk causes gas in people who cannot digest lactose, the sugar present in milk. This is called *lactose intolerance*. It affects about 6% of Australians and is more common in women than men. It occurs in a much greater percentage of certain groups of people including Australian aborigines, Chinese, some people from Middle Eastern countries and some Italians and Greeks. Most of these people have not included dairy products which contain lactose in their diet after weaning and they stop producing the enzyme lactase which is needed to digest lactose.

With lactose intolerance, undigested lactose ferments, causing pain, bloating and diarrhoea. In those people who continue to produce lactase, 90-100% of the lactose they consume is absorbed in the small intestine. In those with lactose intolerance, 25-60% of the lactose is absorbed. The rest passes to the colon where it ferments and causes gas.

Milk (regular and skim), ice cream and some yoghurts contain lactose. Cream, butter and cheese have almost no lactose. A small amount of milk, for example, added to tea or coffee, will not cause problems for those with lactose intolerance. The quantity of lactose in half a cup of milk, for example, is insufficient to generate much gas. Larger quantities of milk in a glass of milk or several scoops of ice cream, may cause symptoms.

Most Anglo-Saxons produce lactase throughout life and have no problems with the lactose in milk. However, some older people—possibly 30%—gradually produce less lactase and find large quantities of milk give them abdominal discomfort and gas.

The easiest solution is for those who are lactose-intolerant to consume less milk and ice cream or to use low-lactose milks or to restrict their dairy products to cheeses. You can also buy enzyme preparations to break down the lactose—usually as drops or tablets to add to milk.

After a bout of gastroenteritis, many infants have a temporary decrease in the enzyme lactase. They may need to avoid milk for a week or two but they do not need to avoid it permanently.

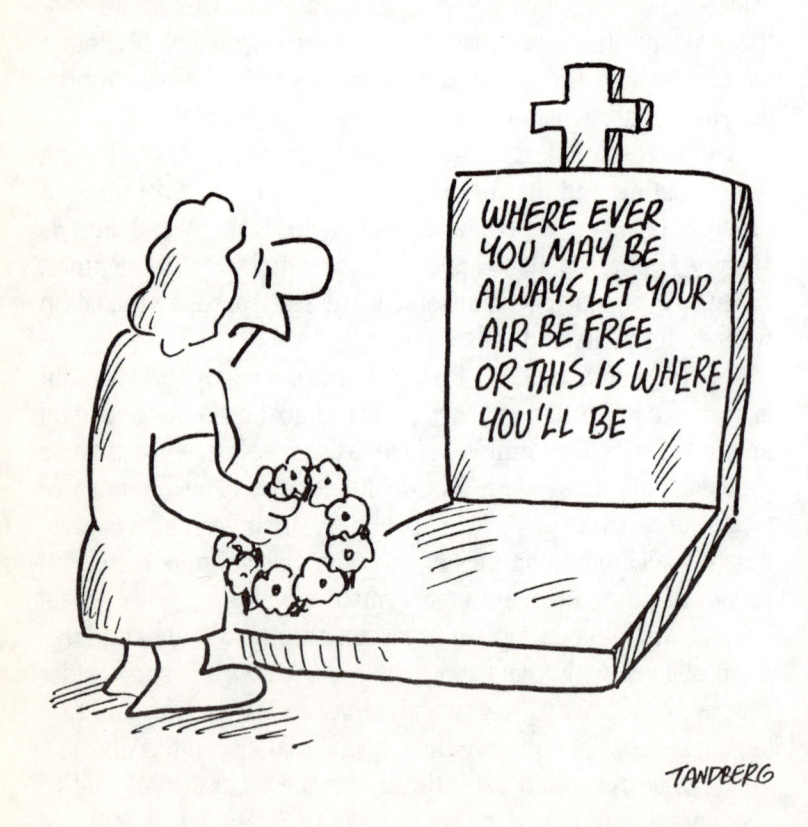

Is yoghurt less likely than milk to cause gas?

Some types of yoghurt are tolerated better than milk. It depends on the bacteria used to thicken the yoghurt and whether they are alive in the product you buy or have been destroyed by pasteurisation. Live strains of some bacteria will partially digest the lactose in yoghurt. This is useful for those with lactose intolerance and will lead to less gas being produced than with milk. Some older people also seem to tolerate yoghurt better than milk. Yoghurt is at least as good a source of calcium as milk.

Some stools sink; others float. It was once believed that floating stools contained a high proportion of fat and were a sign of poor fat digestion. This theory is now known to be wrong. Floating stools contain a lot of gas, not fat. Anyone on a high fibre diet, and particularly those who produce a lot of methane, tend to have floating stools. They are not a sign of digestive problems.

Does sugar cause gas?

Common sugars such as sucrose (cane sugar), maltose (in malted milk), glucose (in fruits, vegetables and glucose drinks), fructose (in fruits and honey) and lactose (in milk) are usually digested by enzymes in the small intestine and should not cause gas.

However, if you lack an enzyme that digests a particular sugar, it will go through to the colon and be fermented by bacteria, causing gas. As mentioned earlier deficiency of lactase after weaning is common in many groups of people (though rare in Anglo-Saxons). A deficiency of any of the other sugar-digesting enzymes is rare and is an inherited problem usually detected in infancy.

How can fruit juices cause gas when they have no fibre?

Fruits and juices contain fructose (fruit sugar) plus some glucose. Some fruits and juices also contain sorbitol, a sugar-alcohol that can cause gas, especially if you consume a large quantity of fruits or juices. This is why apple juice can cause gas and pains in the tummy in young children. Pear juice may have a similar effect. The combination of fructose and sorbitol produces more gas than either substance taken alone.

Apple, pear, grape and prune juices produce gas. Orange, apricot and pineapple juices are less likely to do so.

> 'Vegetarianism is harmless enough but apt to fill a man with self-righteousness and wind'.

What is sorbitol and does it cause gas?

Sorbitol is a sugar alcohol which is present naturally in some fruits and juices, especially apples, pears, cherries, apricots and plums. It is also added to some foods as a sweetener and to give bulk and moisture to carbohydrate-modified jams, sweets and sugarless chewing gum which normally get their bulk from regular sugar. Sorbitol is also added to some cough syrups and medications. If added, it carries the number 420. If present naturally, you have no easy way of knowing.

Very little sorbitol is digested in the small intestine. Most is fermented by bacteria in the bowel, producing gas. In large quantities, sorbitol can cause a lot of gas and also diarrhoea. The high content of sorbitol in apple juice is a major cause of diarrhoea in small children.

The combination of sorbitol and fructose (the sugar found in fruits and honey) causes excessive gas in some people. Apple juice, pear juice (used in many canned fruits whose label says 'in natural fruit juice'), and eating large quantities of apples, pears, cherries or plums may, therefore, cause excess gas in some people.

'A fabis abstinetes' (translates as *Eat no beans*). Pythagoras.

What is mannitol and does it cause gas too?

Mannitol is another sugar alcohol (like sorbitol). It is used in some low calorie products such as jellies and sweets. (Additive number 421.) It is not digested in the small intestine but goes to the bowel where it ferments and causes gas. In large quantities, it also causes diarrhoea.

> 'The foods of the animal kingdom give nitrogen; an unknown process generates sulphur and phosphorus, and hence those emissions of sulphuretted hydrogen of which the effects are known by everyone, but of which the author is never known'.
> Brillat-Savarin.

Does fruit cause gas?

Fruits contain various valuable types of dietary fibre, including pectin. These are fermented in the colon, producing gas. This should not cause any problems.

Fruits also contain the sugar fructose. In large doses, some people do not absorb fructose well in the small intestine. It therefore passes to the colon where it too is fermented by bacteria, producing a lot of gas. In most cases, it is only by eating large quantities of fruits that any problems arise. Apple and pear juice may also cause problems, because it is easy to consume large quantities. The sorbitol in these products may also add to the gas production, as mentioned earlier.

With flatulence, it is better to give than to receive.

Why do stone fruits cause gas and tummy upsets?

When stone fruits are not quite ripe, they have a higher content of pectin. This helps jam to set but it also causes wind. This is not usually a problem. However, when eagerly awaited stone fruits first come into season, it is easy to eat too many and take in larger quantities of pectin than in the usual diet. Gas production will increase. The new season's fruits may also be a little unripe and so have more pectin.

> 'The wind blowest where it will and thou hearest its sound, but thou knowest not whence it comes'. John 3:8.

Why do unripe bananas cause a lot of gas?

Unripe bananas have a higher content of starch and less sugar than ripe ones. The starch in unripe bananas is not digested in the small intestine and passes to the colon as 'resistant starch'. Bacteria ferment resistant starch fast, producing gas. It is not harmful to eat unripe bananas but they may produce a lot of gas and some discomfort in some people. If unripe bananas cause you symptoms, eat only ripe ones.

> If humans let off the 12L of hydrogen that enters the colon each day, the explosion hazard would extend beyond the gas passer to anyone in the general vicinity. The way the bowel disposes of hydrogen is therefore of more than passing interest.

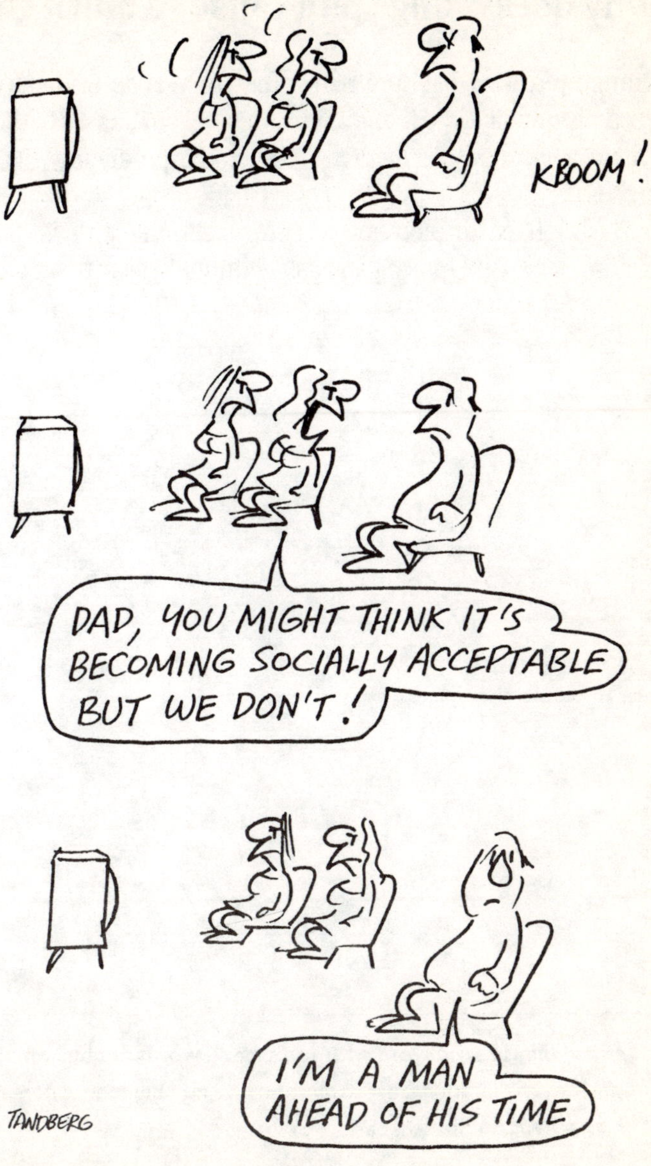
KBOOM!
DAD, YOU MIGHT THINK IT'S BECOMING SOCIALLY ACCEPTABLE BUT WE DON'T!
I'M A MAN AHEAD OF HIS TIME
TANDBERG

Why does orange pith cause so much gas?

Orange pith and peel are rich in pectin, a type of dietary fibre. Pectin is not digested in the small intestine but passes to the colon where it is totally fermented by bacteria, producing gas in the process.

The high pectin content of citrus peel and pith is useful in making jams and marmalade as pectin makes jams set well.

'A man may break a word with you sir; and words are but wind; Ay, and break it in your face, so he break it not behind.' *Comedy of Errors*, William Shakespeare.

Do you get more gas if you eat meat?

Meat is digested in the small intestine and does not increase gases. Meat, poultry and fish produce a lower volume of gas than most other foods.

However, some substances in meat called indoles and skatoles pass to the bowel and may produce smelly gases. Meats empty slowly from the stomach (up to four hours) and then take some hours to be digested in the small intestine. But there is no truth to the idea that meat takes days to be digested and therefore 'rots' and causes an increase in gas. Only someone with a rare disease of the pancreas will fail to digest meat in the small intestine.

'We have, as it were, brought forth wind'. Isaiah.

Do eggs cause gas?

Egg white contains a lot of sulphur in a protein called ovalbumen. When egg white is cooked, some of the sulphur is freed and reacts with hydrogen to form hydrogen sulphide. In small doses this gives cooked eggs their characteristic, and not unpleasant, smell. In large quantities, hydrogen sulphide has the odour of 'rotten eggs'. After eating an egg, you are unlikely to notice any change in gas or smell. If you eat a lot of eggs, you may produce more smelly gas but you will not produce a large volume of gas from eating eggs.

> 'For the gentle wind doth move
> Silently, invisibly'. Blake.

Do fatty foods cause more gas?

Yes, fatty foods are digested in the small intestine to form fatty acids. To neutralise this acid, extra bicarbonate is released in the small intestine. The acid and the bicarbonate form carbon dioxide gas. This can cause discomfort.

Fatty foods also delay the emptying of the stomach. This time lag can increase the unpleasant symptoms associated with flatulence.

Fatty foods include most fast foods, fried foods (especially hot chips which have often been fried twice and soak up an equal amount of fat with each frying), chocolate, cakes, pies and pastries, croissants, biscuits, fatty meats (especially sausages, salami and large fatty steaks), margarine, butter, cream, oils and mayonnaise.

Do different food combinations create more gas?

There is a popular theory that the body cannot digest protein and carbohydrate foods at the same time. This belief stems from the 1930s when the 'Hay Diet' was popular. Its author believed that carbohydrates needed an alkaline medium for their digestion and therefore should not be combined with any acid foods such as fruits, or with proteins since these stimulate acid production in the stomach. According to these theories, any 'wrong' food combinations cause digestive upsets, increase body weight and lead to excess gas. In fact, these theories are wrong.

The body is well designed to handle combinations of foods and many nutritious foods such as nuts, seeds, grains, legumes (beans and peas) and milk contain both carbohydrate and protein within the one food. There is no problem in digesting these foods. In the acidic environment of the stomach, protein-splitting enzymes begin to digest proteins. The fats and carbohydrate are then digested in the small intestine (which is alkaline) and enzymes here also complete the digestion of the proteins. There is no increased gas by combining foods. The gas which legumes produce is not due to their combination of proteins and carbohydrates, but because of the particular type of carbohydrates (oligosaccharides) they contain and their high fibre content.

Would you still produce gas if you ate no fibre?

Yes. Mucins from the lining material of the small intestine pass through to the colon and the proteins and carbohydrates in this cast-off material are fermented by bacteria. However, without fibre, you would produce less gas and pass it less often. You wouldn't produce hydrogen or carbon dioxide but there would be little change in the amount of methane you produced. Most of the gas would probably be nitrogen. Without dietary fibre, your bowel would be less healthy and you would be constipated.

Sprouting seeds may reduce their potential for flatulence. Some seeds, however, produce extra oligosaccharides during germination and these may produce more gas when they reach the colon.

Would you still produce gas if you were fasting?

You produce much less gas when you are going without food but you still produce some. You will still swallow air and it will contain nitrogen, some of which will reach the colon. You will not produce hydrogen or carbon dioxide as these gases come from fermentation of dietary fibre and resistant starch in the diet. However, the intestine will still produce mucins, the lining of the intestine will continue to shed dead cells (a little like moulting) and bacteria in the colon will die. Each of these provides food for live bacteria to ferment and this will produce gases.

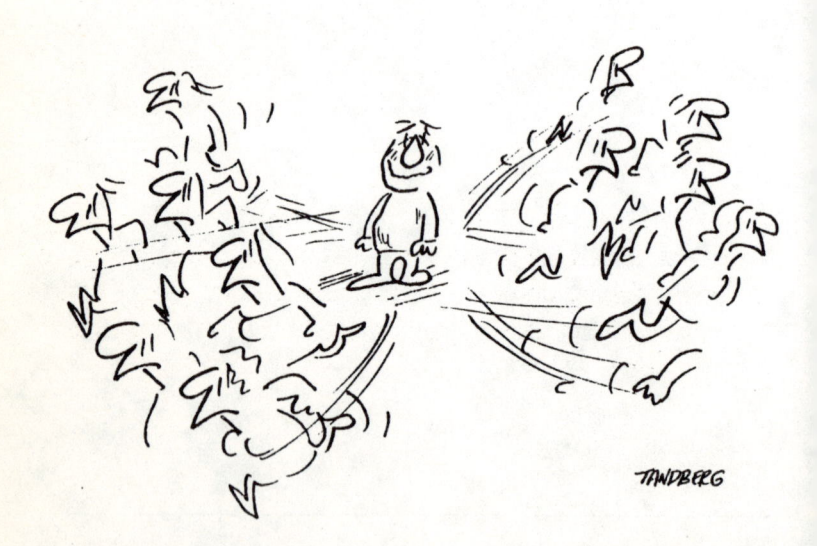

Why does gas sometimes smell unpleasant?

About 99% of the gases produced are odourless gases such as hydrogen, methane and carbon dioxide. Any odour associated with gas comes from small amounts of volatile substances. These include hydrogen sulphide, mercaptans, indole, skatole and methyl sulphides as well as other substances which have not yet been identified. The nose can sense these odours in concentrations as low as one part in 100 million! Highly qualified 'sniffers' would be needed to distinguish between the various aromas. Most people with such 'noses' tend to work in either of the more rewarding and socially acceptable industries of perfume or wine.

Most people are familiar with the classical smell of rotten egg gas, or hydrogen sulphide. Only those with sulphate-reducing bacteria in their colon can produce this gas. However, the other half of the population without these bacteria will still pass volatile (and smelly) by-products of protein digestion, including indole and skatole. Meat eaters may produce more of these substances than vegetarians.

Some spices, herbs, especially asafoetida (a pungent-smelling herb from a member of the fennel family, used in many Indian dishes), garlic and onions and dried shrimp pastes (used in many Asian dishes) also give off pungent and strong-smelling gases.

Does smelly gas indicate disease in the intestine?

Pungent odours are rarely due to any disease in the bowel. Aroma is usually due to what you eat. For example, garlic, onions, eggplant, mushrooms and a wide variety of herbs and Asian spices may produce smelly gases. In most cases, the situation rights itself quickly.

In some rare cases, pungent odours occur when the pancreas is not functioning normally so that proteins are not digested in the small intestine and pass instead to the colon where they ferment and produce a number of nasty-smelling sulphur-containing compounds.

Pungent, smelly gases in flatus can arise from bleeding in the gastrointestinal tract, for example, from a bleeding peptic ulcer. Small amounts of blood from a polyp or bowel cancer do not cause these same pungent gases. If the odour of flatus changes, it is usually due to something you have eaten. If the change in smell persists, there may be some disease in the bowel and you should see your doctor.

'May the wind be always at your back'.

Can intestinal gas cause bad breath?

Substances produced in the colon can be reabsorbed into the blood and pass to the lungs and out the mouth. Some of these can smell unpleasant on the breath. 'Garlic breath' is a good example of this. Some garlic breath comes from the stomach but some comes later when the garlic releases sulphur compounds in the colon. This may explain why garlic breath is present long after the garlic has left the stomach.

The dog's sense of smell is 10,000 times more sensitive than a human's. This olfactory ability could provide an important tool for research into gas. Perhaps we could look forward to another breed of research assistant: bloodhound diagnostic researchers, certified by olfactory board examinations.

When your tummy bloats after meals, is this due to gas?

Distension of the abdomen occurs in people with a condition known as irritable bowel syndrome. The abdomen is usually flattest in the morning and gets progressively bigger during the day, especially after meals. Some special tests have shown that this distension is not due to gas. It may be due to changes in the elastic qualities or tone of the muscles of the intestine. If these muscles become less elastic they may be more easily blown up by an amount of gas which is usually considered normal.

Most women have an abdomen which is convex rather than concave. In spite of their dislike of this 'tummy', it is quite normal and is not a case of 'bloating'.

A true bloated or distended abdomen is something beyond the normal limits and the increased measurements in girth are greater than normally occurs with progressive eating during the day. True bloating occurs more commonly in women and those who suffer from it may feel so uncomfortable that they need to undo their belt or change to looser clothing at the end of the day, even when they have not overeaten.

'This too shall pass . . . ' Nathaniel Hawthorne.

'The wind bloweth where it wills'. Gospel According to St Luke.

Why do women with anorexia feel so bloated?

Women who have anorexia nervosa often complain of bloating and abdominal pain if they eat even a small amount of food. With their haphazard eating, the movement of the gut contents slows down. The rectum may also become distended and, by reflex, this slows emptying of the stomach and increases the feeling of fullness and bloating.

Anorexia nervosa is also characterised by extreme thinness. Without a normal covering of fat and with poor muscle tone from semi-starvation, the abdomen tends to protrude more than you would expect in a lean woman. Any time an anorexic woman does eat, she is very conscious that her usually empty intestine now has some contents. Most anorexic women, with their intense fear of fat, see this as 'bloating'.

Saint Jerome forbad his nuns to eat beans, believing that *in partibus genitalibus titillationes producunt* (translates as *They tickle the genitals*).

How can gas be measured?

Measuring gas can be difficult. Collection of gas from the anus is neither comfortable nor foolproof. The tip of a flexible rubber tube is inserted into the anus and taped in place. The tube is connected to a gas bag. The possibility of leakage was solved by two volunteers who lay in a warm bath for an hour, checking to see if they could detect any bubbling as gas collected in the bag. The method appeared to work. However, both tube and bag must be removed for a bowel motion and replaced as soon as practicable.

The other more complicated method is to place subjects in a small airtight room equipped with an airlock. Fresh air is passed through the room at a known rate and the excretion of hydrogen can be measured as the difference between the out-flow and in-flow concentrations. The amount of hydrogen in expired air can also be measured so the amount of hydrogen passed as flatus can be calculated from the difference between the total hydrogen being excreted and the amount of hydrogen on the breath.

An X-ray of the abdomen is another method that can measure the area of gas bubbles present but it does not always correlate with symptoms of gas.

It is much easier to measure gases expired on the breath. For example, the amount of hydrogen in expired air is measured using a device similar to a breathalyser used to measure alcohol. Breath hydrogen tests are used to measure fermentation of sugars such as lactose (milk sugar). Most people of Anglo-Saxon origin and from some parts of Africa, digest lactose in the small intestine. Most other people throughout the world do not, and the undigested lactose reaches the colon where it is fermented and produces a lot of hydrogen. This is called lactose intolerance and the rise in breath hydrogen after drinking milk can be used to diagnose it.

The same principle can be used to measure if other sugars such as sucrose (ordinary cane sugar) or fructose (fruit sugar) and related substances such as sorbitol are passing through the small intestine without being digested. Any increase in breath hydrogen suggests that the sugar is not being digested.

> 'The wind whirleth about continually, and the wind returneth according to the circuits'. Ecclesiastes.

Why does your tummy rumble?

Your stomach is more likely to rumble or gurgle when it is empty and you are hungry. The thought, sight or smell of food stimulates the digestive juices and triggers muscular contractions of the stomach, small intestine and bowel. The contents of the intestine are a mixture of fluid and gas so the turbulence created by the movements produces the noises. They may seem quite loud but other people will not notice them as much as you think.

You may also notice noises from the upper part of the gastrointestinal tract if you swallow a lot of air while eating and drinking.

Noises from further down—in the colon—come from gases in the colon. They are usually worse if you are trying to stop gas escaping.

> I sat next to the Duchess at tea
> It was just as I feared it would be
> Her rumblings abdominal
> Were simply phenomenal
> But everyone thought it was me.

Why does my stomach rumble soon after eating a Chinese meal?

Carbohydrate foods such as rice and vegetables (the main components of many Chinese meals) pass through the stomach quickly, especially if eaten without significant quantities of protein or fat. This means your stomach is empty soon after eating these foods and it will give a hunger rumble to ask for more food. A meal of fruit will have a similar effect. Proteins delay the emptying of the stomach to some extent and a meal or snack which is high in fat will take the longest time to empty. Including some protein or fat in a meal therefore stops you feeling hungry and having a rumbling stomach too soon after a meal.

Can you stop your tummy rumbling?

You will have fewer tummy rumbles if you eat small frequent meals. Once the rumbles or gurgles start, try to eat something. If they seem to be coming from the lower end of the intestine, there is nothing much you can do about it although passing wind will help.

What causes burps?

Belching or burping is a way to get rid of gas from the stomach. This may come from air swallowed while eating, air swallowed just before a burp or from air incorporated into foods.

If you are tense, anxious or feeling stressed, you are more likely to swallow air without realising it. Stressed people often complain of having lots of gas.

Fizzy drinks produce gas in the stomach, mainly from the carbon dioxide they contain. Some of this is burped and the rest is absorbed from the intestine or passes through the bowel.

Other 'airy' foods such as pavlova, whipped desserts or whipped toppings, or even ice cream which has a lot of air whipped into it, also increase gas. These foods may make you burp more.

> 'All citizens shall be allowed to pass gas whenever necessary'.
> Claudius.

Does burping or belching help get rid of gas?

Belching (colloquially called 'burping') occurs when gas is ejected noisily through the mouth. Gas in the stomach may make you feel full and bloated and belching gets rid of some of this gas. However, when you burp deliberately, you will unconsciously swallow air just before you burp and the burp does not get rid of as much air as you swallow. This means that any relief from deliberate burping is short-lived.

The air you swallow contains **oxygen** and **nitrogen**. All the oxygen is absorbed from the stomach and the first part of the small intestine. There is no oxygen present beyond that point.

Two thirds of the nitrogen in swallowed air is absorbed into the blood and is excreted on the breath. The remaining third is passed from the anus.

Onions and garlic contain sulphur compounds which add an aroma to gases emerging at either end of the gastrointestinal tract.

When someone burps, are they showing a lack of manners or could they try harder to suppress the burp?

Sometimes gas in the upper part of the intestine is due to heartburn when acid refluxes into the oesophagus and irritates it. Burping often gives relief.

At other times, burping is a habit and is related either to swallowing air or to stress. These types of burps disappear when the person is concentrating on something. They may return when they lose interest and are bored or stressed again.

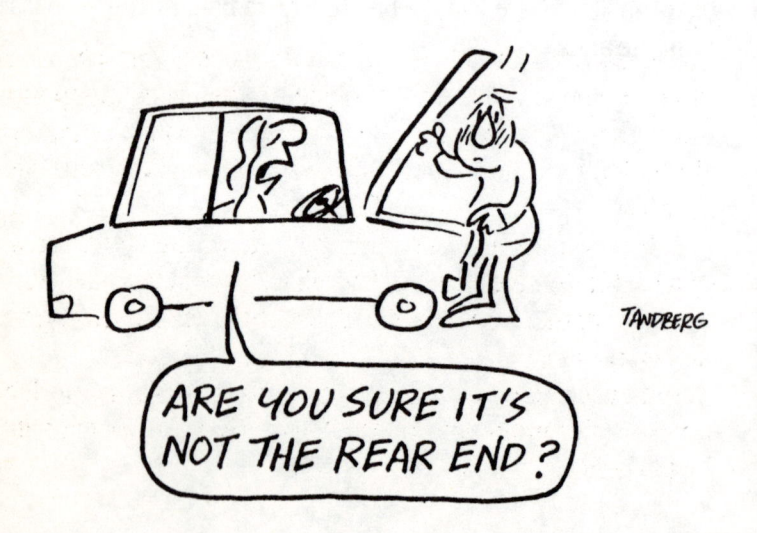

Is it harmful to suppress a burp?

No. You can either burp air you swallow when eating or drinking or it can be absorbed from the intestine or pass through the bowel. If you suppress a burp, you may feel full and uncomfortable for a while until the stomach empties its contents into the small intestine. This may take a couple of hours, especially if the meal contained fats.

Why do you have to 'burp' babies?

When babies suck, they swallow air. This forms gas in the stomach and is relieved by bringing up the bubble (burping). If a large amount of gas is brought up, some food may come with the air bubble. This is not the same as vomiting and is no cause for alarm.

Babies swallow more air when they are very hungry at the start of a feed, if they are sucking through a teat with too small a hole, or from a mother with retracted nipples, or if they are sucking from an empty bottle.

Some babies have quite severe reflux of food. This may be due to a weak valve in the lower oesophagus, often associated with a hiatus hernia.

Is infant colic due to gas?

Swallowing air may cause colic with attacks of severe abdominal pain. Colic sometimes occurs with underfeeding, nasal obstruction or too small a hole in a teat.

Possetting, or regurgitating small mouthfuls of milk, is common, especially in breast-fed babies who get their milk too fast or swallow too much air while being fed.

Do you swallow more air with food or drinks?

Generally you swallow more air with drinks than with foods. On average, each swallow puts 2–3 mL of air into the stomach. The volume may be greater with liquids.

'A rushing mighty wind'. The Acts of the Apostles.

Do you swallow more air when drinking through a straw?

Many people do, so if you want to impress a special friend, throw away the straw.

> 'It is universally well known, that in digesting our common food, there is created or produced in the bowels of human creatures, a great quantity of wind. That the permitting of this air to escape and mix with the atmosphere, is usually offensive to the company, from the fetid smell that accompanies it. That all well-bred people therefore, to avoid giving offence, forcibly restrain the efforts of nature to discharge that wind. That so retained contrary to nature, it not only gives frequently present great pain, but occasions future diseases such as habitual cholics, ruptures, tympanies &c, often destructive of the constitution and sometimes life itself.
>
> Were it not for the odiously offensive smell accompanying such escapes, polite people would probably be under no more restraint in discharging such wind in company, than they are in spitting or in blowing their noses.
>
> My prize question therefore should be: To discover some drug, wholesome and not disagreeable, to be mixed with our common food or sauces, that shall render the natural discharges of wind from our bodies not only inoffensive, but agreeable as perfumes.'
> *Benjamin Franklin's proposal to the Royal Academy in Brussels, 1770.*

Do you swallow more air when drinking from a can?

Yes. When drinking liquids, it is possible to swallow up to twice the volume of air as liquid. This happens with a 'glug, glug' type of fast drinking, often from a bottle or can. Much of the air escapes by burping. The common practice of some young men in drinking a whole can of liquid and then producing a loud burp comes from swallowing a lot of air with this style of consumption.

Why do you get hiccups?

Hiccups come from a repeated and involuntary spasm of muscles of the diaphragm which separate the chest from the abdomen. The most common cause is irritation of the diaphragm by an over-full stomach. Sometimes hiccups are due to an inflammation in that area, an ulcer or pleurisy affecting the diaphragm. Some serious diseases such as kidney failure can also cause hiccups. Mostly there is no obvious cause.

How can you stop hiccups?

Hiccups usually stop spontaneously. There are also a number of unproven remedies to stop them such as getting a fright, a slap on the back, standing on your head, or trying to drink out of the wrong side of a glass. The most effective treatment is to find the cause.

Euphemisms for 'fart'

Backfire
Beef heart
Botty-banger
Braff
Break wind
Breezer
Burp
Cough
Down wind
Drop a bundle
Drop your lunch
Fluff
Go off
Let off
Let one fly
Lunch
Make a smell
Raspberry tart
Shoot a fairy
Silent but deadly (used by American teenagers in the 1950s)
Squeaker
Tiparillo
Windy Pop

Glossary

Aerophagy: Swallowing or sucking in air, either voluntarily or subconsciously.

Anal canal: Passage leading from the rectum.

Aroma: The smell associated with the emission of flatus. Categorised as mild to pungent, and, to some, repugnant. Not to be confused with aromatherapy.

Bile: A bitter, greenish-yellow fluid made in the liver and stored in the gall bladder between meals. With eating, the gall bladder contracts and empties bile into the small intestine to help digest fats.

Bloating: Uncomfortable distension of the upper abdomen, usually after a meal. Often associated with nausea.

Borborygmi: Audible sounds coming from the mixture of fluid and gas in the stomach or large bowel. Muscular contractions in the bowel wall increase the symphony of sound.

Bowel, large: Also known as the *large intestine* or *colon*. Begins at the caeum and appendix on the right side of the abdomen and finishes at the rectum. Total length is 1.5–2 metres.

Bowel, small: Also known as the *small intestine*. Includes the area between the duodenum and the caecum. Major site of all food digestion and absorption of nutrients. Smaller in diameter than the large bowel and about 6 metres long. Inner surface is lined with innumerable tiny finger-like villi which increase the area available to absorb nutrients to something the size of a tennis court.

Break wind: An expression used in the 16th century to describe both belching and farting.

Burbulence: A term used to cover aerophagy, belching, bloating, borborygmi, burping, distension, flatulence, flatus and wind.

Burp: To belch out wind from the stomach.

Caecum: Beginning of the large bowel. Contents from the small intestine enter the caecum at the ileo-caecal valve.

Candida: Types of yeasts. About half the population has various species of candida in the mouth, where they do no harm. After treatment with antibiotics, with immunodeficiency (HIV infections) and in severe conditions such as cancer, the yeast may flourish. Possible problems include infection in the mouth (especially likely in babies and very old people), vagina and oesophagus. Candida is often blamed for bowel disturbances and poor health but is rarely the true culprit.

Carbohydrate: Compounds of carbon, hydrogen and oxygen. Most carbohydrates have twice as much hydrogen as oxygen as occurs in water—giving them the name 'hydrate of carbon'. Includes sugars, starches and some types of dietary fibre.

Carbohydrate, complex: Carbohydrates made up of many glucose units joined together. Also called 'starch'.

Colon: *see Bowel, large*

Colonic: Relating to the colon.

Colitis: Inflammation of the colon. Occurs with ulcerative colitis and Crohn's disease.

Constipation: Infrequent passage of small hard bowel motions. Related to the consistency of the faeces rather than the frequency.

Distension: Swelling of the abdomen 'like a balloon'. May occur in the lower area of the abdomen, in the upper abdomen under the rib cage or be generalised over the whole abdomen.

Diverticula: Small 'blow outs' or 'pockets' which can occur at weak spots in the colon, especially on the left side. Commonly associated with a low fibre diet.

Donor: One who emits flatus, either overtly or surreptitiously.

Down wind: Suggested to move up wind. Euphemism for fart.

Duodenum: The first section of the small bowel or small intestine.

Enzyme: Protein catalysts which help biochemical reactions take place and split complex substances into more simple ones. For example, lactase is an enzyme that splits lactose (milk sugar) into its component sugars of glucose and galactose.

Eructate: To belch out, especially wind from the stomach.

Faeces: Waste matter excreted from the rectum via the anal canal. By weight, faeces consists of 75% water and 25% solids—half dietary fibre and half bacteria.

Farting: Passing gas. Ranging from surreptitious to flamboyant judged on volume and aroma, from odourless to repugnant.

Fermentation: A reaction carried out by microorganisms in the absence of oxygen. In the colon, bacteria ferment most types of dietary fibre as well as any carbohydrates or proteins which reach the colon.

Flatoanalysis: The determination of the nature of intestinal gases.

Flatogram: A chart documenting the number and times gas is passed by farting or belching. Similar to a temperature chart. Not commonly used, but potentially useful.

Flatology: The scientific study of intestinal gases.

Flatological: Adjective of flatology.

Flatogenic: Foods likely to produce excessive gas.

Flatometry: The science of measuring flatus.

Flatulation: The act of expelling gas from the anus.

Flatulence: From the Latin *flatulentus, flatus*—a blowing.

Flatus: Passage of gas.

Fructose: A sugar found in fruits and honey. When combined with glucose, it forms the sugar sucrose (cane sugar). Both fructose and sucrose are normally digested in the small intestine. In large doses, or when combined with sorbitol, some fructose enters the colon where it is fermented and may cause a lot of gas.

Gastrointestinal tract: Sometimes called the GI tract or the 'gut'. Extends from mouth to the anus. Includes oesophagus, stomach, small intestine (duodenum, jejunum and ileum) and the large intestine (colon and rectum). Total length is about 9 metres.

Ileum: The last (or *distal*) third of the small intestine.

Indole: A smelly gas released in flatus. Comes from the breakdown of tryptophan, one of the amino acids found in proteins. Used in very small doses in perfumes but in larger quantities, contributes to the unpleasant odour of faeces.

Lactase: An enzyme produced in the small intestine to break down lactose, the sugar in milk, to its component sugars, glucose and galactose. Mammals, except for some humans, do not produce lactase after weaning. Some humans also fail to produce enough lactase to break down the sugar in large quantities of milk. The lactose then passes to the colon where it ferments, producing gas. The sea lion is the only mammal that doesn't produce lactose.

Lactose: The main sugar in the milk of mammals, including human milk. Consists of one molecule of glucose joined to one of a sugar called galactose.

Large intestine: *see Bowel, large*

Mannitol: A sugar alcohol substance added to foods as a sweetener and to stop them becoming dry. Not digested in the small intestine but fermented in the colon, producing gas. Large doses cause diarrhoea.

Mercaptans: Another smelly product released in flatus. Comes from the digestion of sulphur-containing amino acids in proteins. Bacteria in the colon ferment mercaptans to produce methane and hydrogen sulphide gases. The hydrogen sulphide has the odour of 'rotten eggs'.

Methane: An odourless gas also known as 'marsh gas' because it forms in marshes (along with smelly gases such as ammonia and hydrogen sulphide). Produced in the left side of the colon by those who have certain types of bacteria. Cows and other ruminant animals produce much larger volumes of methane.

Mucins: A complex layer of lining material in the intestine made up of protein and several types of carbohydrate. Contains important proteins or immunoglobulins needed for defence against infection and allergy.

Oesophagus: The gullet or tube connecting the mouth with the stomach.

Oligosaccharides: Carbohydrates with 3-15 sugar units. Some oligosaccharides in legumes (dried beans and peas) are not digested in the small intestine and are fermented in the colon, producing a lot of gas.

Passive farting: Exposure to surreptitious flatus emission by persons (or dogs) nearby, usually in confined spaces.

Pectin: A type of dietary fibre present in fruit, especially unripe fruit and citrus peel.

Raffinose: An oligosaccharide found in dried beans.

Recipient: One exposed to aromatic gas emitted by a donor, usually unrequested. Origin of the expression 'it is better to give than to receive'.

Rectum: The last 15-20 centimetres of the large bowel. Acts as a reservoir for faeces.

Reflux: The passage of gut contents in the reverse direction, for example, acid reflux from the stomach into the oesophagus, or the contents of the caecum into the ileum through the ileocaecal valve.

Resistant starch: Starch (or complex carbohydrate) that resists being digested by enzymes called amylases in the small intestine and passes through to the colon where it is fermented by bacteria, producing valuable acids—and gas. The method of cooking, cooling and processing foods determines whether their starches are digested by amylases or become resistant starch.

Short chain fatty acids: Also known as volatile fatty acids. Includes acetic, propionic and butyric acids produced in the colon by bacterial fermentation of complex carbohydrates and some types of dietary fibre.

Skatole: An unpleasant smelling gas released in flatus. Like indole, skatole comes from the breakdown of tryptophan, an amino acid component of protein foods.

Small intestine: *see Bowel, small*

Sorbitol: A sugar alcohol used as a sweetener. Also a natural substance in apples and apple juice. A small part of the sorbitol in food is converted to fructose. The rest is fermented by bacteria in the colon, producing gas. Large doses may cause diarrhoea.

Stachyose: An oligosaccharide found in dried beans.

Starch: *see Carbohydrate, complex*

Stool: Faeces. Waste matter excreted from the rectum through the anal canal.

Sulphates: Salts of sulphuric acid.

Sulphides: Compounds containing sulphur and an element with a positive charge.

Sulphites: Salts of sulphurous acid.

Transit: The time taken for food and fluid to pass through the length of the intestine, from mouth to anus. It involves several stages. Gastric emptying from the stomach may be quick with liquids and slower with solids. Fruit eaten on its own empties fast. A normal meal takes about 4 hours to empty completely from the stomach. The transit time for some of the food eaten to pass from the mouth to the caecum may be as fast as 15 minutes but usually takes from 1-2 hours. Transit time through the colon takes the longest time, from 24-36 hours.

Smell of gunpowder: A euphemism for a smelly fart, first used in the late 19th century in the British army and relating to the analogy with the explosion from a cannon.

Up wind: Desirable position (*see* down wind).

Verbascose: An oligosaccharide found in beans. Not related to verbosity, although similarly producing an amount of (hot) air.

Index

acetic acid 24
acid 1
   stomach 7
alcohol 3
altitude 7, 30
amino acids 24, 25
ammonia 25
anorexia nervosa 67
antibiotics 28
anticholinergic drugs 28
anus 21
anxiety 13
apple juice 49, 50
apricot juice 49
aroma 14, 64, 73
artichokes 29
asafoetida 63
astronauts 30

babies 9, 75
bacteria 4, 6, 7, 14, 23, 27, 33, 47, 52, 62
bad breath 65
bananas 54
beans 27, 29, 31, 38, 40
   green 42
   soya 41, 42
beer 24
belching 7, 72, 73
bile 3
bleeding 64
bloating 11, 28, 34, 35, 45, 66, 73
bowel cancer 26, 39, 64
bread 24, 44
breath hydrogen tests 68
breathalysers 68
broccoli 38, 43
Brussels sprouts 38, 43
burping 7, 28, 29, 34, 36, 44, 72, 73, 74, 75, 78, 81
butter 45

cabbage 6, 24, 38, 43
caecum 4
calcium 28, 47

candida 44
candidiasis 44
carbohydrate-modified jams 50
carbohydrates 3, 4, 60, 71
   complex 1, 3, 6
carbon dioxide 7, 13, 18, 23, 24, 30, 40, 59, 61, 63, 72
carbonated beverages 31
cauliflower 38, 43
charcoal, activated 28
cheese 28, 38, 45
chewing 1
chewing gum 50
children 9, 23
   diarrhoea in 50
Chinese meals 71
chips 24
cider 24
colic 76
colitis 28
colon 3, 4, 7
complex carbohydrates 1, 3, 6
constipation 4, 17, 35, 61
cosmonauts 30
cream 45
Crohn's disease 26
cystic fibrosis 26

dairy products 45
diarrhoea 5, 35, 45, 50, 51
   in children 50
dietary fibre 3, 4, 5, 6, 7, 23, 28, 38, 39, 40, 56
digestion 1
digestive juices 70
digestive system 1, 2
distension 10, 17, 20, 35, 66
diverticular disease 26
dried fruits 24
duodenum 7

eggplant 64
eggs 58
elderly 12
enzymes 1, 40, 60
euphemisms for 'fart' 80

faeces 4, 5
fart 10
fasting 6, 62
fat 3, 14, 71
fatty acids 8, 12
   short chain 27, 39
fatty foods 59
fennel 63
fermentation 4, 8, 14, 27, 42, 52, 68
fizzy drinks 72
flatulence 59
flatus 8, 10, 15, 27, 68
food combining 25, 60
fried foods 59
fructans 15
fructose 15, 48, 49, 52, 69
fruits 52, 53, 71
fullness 3

galactopinitol 40
gall bladder 3
gall stones 34
garlic 24, 38, 63, 64, 65, 73
gas 6, 7, 11
gas, measurement of 68
gas, production of 10, 13
gas, volume of 4, 10, 11, 16, 22, 35
   in men 16, 23
   in women 16, 23
gases, smelly 14, 23, 57, 58, 63, 64
gastroenteritis 46
glucose 48, 49
grape juice 49
greenhouse gases 18
gurgles 70

haemorrhoids 19
Hay Diet 60
heartburn 36, 74
herbs 63, 64
hiatus hernia 36, 75
hiccups 79
honey 50
hormone replacement therapy 17
hormones 16
hunger 3
hydrogen 7, 13, 16, 23, 24, 27, 32, 33, 54, 61, 63, 68
   breath tests for 68
hydrogen sulphide 23, 27, 43, 58, 63

ice cream 28, 45
idli 42
indole 57, 63
infants 46, 76
inulin 29
irritable bowel syndrome 11, 35, 66

jams 50
juices 24, 50
   fruit 49

lactase 45
lactose 38, 45, 48, 68
lactose intolerance 28, 29, 45, 68
large intestine 4
leeks 38
legumes 41
lignin 4

maltose 48
manganese 41
manninotriose 40
mannitol 51
meat 14, 57
men 16, 23
mercaptans 43, 63
methane 7, 16, 18, 23, 26, 27, 32, 33, 47, 61, 63
methyl sulphides 43, 63
milk 28, 38, 45, 69
mood 33
mountaineers 30
mucins 61, 62
mushrooms 64
mustard seeds 40, 41

nitrogen 7, 13, 24, 61, 73
noise 19

odour 7, 16, 43
oesophagus 1, 36, 74
oligosaccharides 27, 40, 41, 42, 60, 61
onions 15, 24, 38, 63, 64, 73
orange juice 49
orange peel 56
oxygen 7, 73

pain 20, 31, 35, 37, 45, 76
pancreas 3, 64

pancreatic juice 3
pear juice 49
pectin 52, 53, 56
peptic ulcer 64
pineapple juice 49
pinitol 40
polyp 64
possetting 76
potato crisps 24
potatoes 12
preservatives 24
progestogen 17
protein 1, 3, 14, 24, 25, 60, 63, 64, 71
prune juice 49
Pujol, Joseph 25

raffinose 27, 40, 41, 42
rectum 4, 10, 22
reflux 1, 75
regurgitation 76
resistant starch 54, 62
rice 71
rotten egg gas 63
rumblings 70, 71, 72

saliva 1
scuba divers 31
seeds 38
  mustard 40, 41
  sprouting 61
short chain fatty acids 27, 39
shrimp 63
skatole 57, 63
small intestine 3, 4, 7
smelly gases 14, 23, 57, 58, 63, 64
sodium metabisulphite 24
sorbitol 49, 50, 69
soya beans 40, 41
soya milk 28
spices 14, 29, 63, 64
sprouting 41, 61

stachyose 27, 40, 42
starch 1, 4, 8, 23, 27, 54
  resistant 54, 62
stomach 1, 2, 3, 7
stomach acid 1, 36
stools 39
  floating 47
stress 74
sucrose 48, 69
sugars 3, 8, 23, 27, 48
sulphides 23
sulphur 58, 64
sulphur compounds 15, 23, 43, 65, 73
sulphur-containing foods 24
sulphur dioxide 7
swallowed air 1, 7, 9, 24, 38, 62, 75, 76, 77, 78

tempeh 41-2
tension 13, 33, 72
therapies 28
tofu 42
transit time 4, 16, 26
  in men 4, 5
  in women 4, 5
trisulphides 43
turbulence 70
turnips 38, 43

vegetables 29, 71
verbascose 27, 40, 42
vomiting 75

wine 24
women 16, 23

X-ray 68

yeast 44
yoghurt 45, 47